The Best Darn Hyperth

Studies on the Overactive Thyroid Gland

By: James M. Lowrance © 2010

The Best Darn Hyperthyroidism Book!

TABLE OF CONTENTS:

CHAPTER ONE
Hyperthyroidism Basic Facts
Overactive Thyroid Gland General Information
CHAPTER TWO
Major Causes of Hyperthyroidism and Treatments
Common Contributors to Thyrotoxicity
CHAPTER THREE
Graves' Disease Hyperthyroidism and Treatments
Autoimmune Caused Hyperthyroidism
CHAPTER FOUR
Radioactive Iodine Ablation of the Thyroid
Cell Destruction of Diseased Glands
CHAPTER FIVE
Treatment for Hashitoxicosis versus Graves' Disease
Patients with Temporary Hyperthyroidism
CHAPTER SIX
Why Doctors Sometimes Delay Treatment for Hashimoto's Thyroiditis
Problems with Hashitoxicosis

The Best Darn Hyperthyroidism Book!

CHAPTER SEVEN
Manifestations of Thyroid Eye Disease
Autoimmune Eyeball Problems and Their Treatments

CHAPTER EIGHT
Symptoms and Manifestations of Thyroid Storm
The Hyperthyroid Condition Requiring Emergency Care

CHAPTER NINE
My Review of Mary Shomon's Hyperthyroid Book
Another Great Resource for Patients with Hyperthyroidism

CHAPTER TEN
Support for Struggling Thyroid Patients
Two Reasons Why Information and Support Resources are Important

CHAPTER ELEVEN
Coping with Thyroid Disease
Methods for Dealing with a Lifetime Health Disorder

The Best Darn Hyperthyroidism Book!

CHAPTER ONE

Hyperthyroidism Basic Facts

Overactive Thyroid Gland General Information

Hyperthyroid disorders account for approximately 20% of thyroid disorder cases. An overactive thyroid gland can cause an array of symptoms but treatments are available.

Hyperthyroidism is a term meaning a person's bodily metabolism is abnormally sped up due to the T3 and/or T4 thyroid hormone levels increasing too high in the body. Symptoms vary in severity among individuals, according to how advanced hyperthyroidism has become at the time of diagnosis.

Major Causes of Hyperthyroidism

Most cases of hyperthyroidism are caused by Graves' disease, an autoimmune disease of the thyroid gland.

With Grave's, auto-antibodies are sent from the immune system cause stimulation of excessive amounts of thyroid hormone production. Graves' patients experience thyroid gland inflammation and enlargement to varied degrees, referred to as "toxic diffuse goiters". Thyroid autoimmunity is a "primary" cause of an overactive thyroid gland.

Another primary cause of an overactive thyroid gland would include "hot nodules", which are tumorous-growths in the gland that absorb iodine in the body and begin producing thyroid hormone just as normal thyroid tissue does.

A less common "secondary" cause of hyperthyroidism would include excessive intake of iodine which can also act as a trigger for primary thyroid autoimmunity.

Temporary types, of thyroiditis occurring in pregnant women or following giving birth or as a result of viral illnesses that settle in the thyroid gland, will cause a short-term phase of hyperthyroidism.

The Best Darn Hyperthyroidism Book!

Treated hypothyroid patients can become hyperthyroid from taking too high a dose of thyroid hormone replacement, sometimes referred to as "dose induced thyrotoxicity".

Hyperthyroid Symptoms

The symptoms of a sped up metabolism from hyperthyroidism include:

- nervousness and anxiety
- tremor (especially in the hands)
- rapid pulse and breathing
- hypertension
- diarrhea
- oily skin and hair
- increased sweating
- increased hunger and thirst
- changes in menstrual cycle and sex drive
- goiter
- rapid weight loss

Patients with Graves' disease may also experience symptoms of muscle weakness and wasting referred to as "myopathy".

They may also develop an inflammatory condition affecting the eyes called "Graves' Ophthalmopathy" or "Thyroid Eye Disease".

Diagnosis

Blood tests of thyroid hormone levels and/or the TSH level can help to diagnose hyperthyroidism. Thyroid hormones (T4 and T3) will elevate to levels above normal values, while TSH (pituitary hormone) will decrease to levels below normal values. When testing is conducted to determine the cause of hyperthyroidism, blood tests for thyroid antibodies may be ordered to confirm or rule out Graves' disease as the cause.

A Radioactive Iodine Uptake Test (RAIU) might also be performed to determine if the thyroid gland is absorbing high levels of iodine which can indicate that it is overactive. If only a certain area of the gland is absorbing high levels of iodine, this can point to hot nodules and an additional Radioactive Iodine Scan (radiology camera) might also be performed at the same time or separately to further evaluate nodules in the gland.

The Best Darn Hyperthyroidism Book!

Treatment

In some cases of hyperthyroidism, the administering of anti-thyroid drugs designed to slow thyroid hormone production will be the initial treatment and possible the only one needed. Beta-blocker medications that moderate the activity of adrenaline in the body can help to alleviate symptoms and may be combined with anti-thyroid drugs.

Surgical procedures are required in some cases of hot nodules, to remove them or part of the thyroid gland if multi-nodules are present (several). Thyroid removal surgery called "thyroidectomy" may also be needed in cases of Graves' disease that cannot be controlled by drug therapies or the gland may be ablated (destroyed) through administering radioactive iodine in a large enough to dose to kill-out the entire gland. Afterward, patients whose thyroid glands are ablated or removed will require thyroid hormone replacement. This is to treat resulting hypothyroidism, as a lifelong treatment.

The Best Darn Hyperthyroidism Book!

CHAPTER TWO

Major Causes of Hyperthyroidism and Treatments

Common Contributors to Thyrotoxicity

As mentioned previously, approximately 20% of thyroid disease cases are hyperthyroid conditions. There are several causes for overactive thyroid disorders and treatments available for them.

The term "thyrotoxicity" simply means that abnormally high levels of thyroid hormone in the body are causing a toxic reaction also referred to as "hyperthyroidism".

While the majority of hyperthyroid conditions are a result of auto-antibodies that stimulate excessive thyroid hormone levels, there are a number of other causes as addressed in the subheadings that follow.

Temporary Thyroiditis

Some people experiencing viral infections or pregnancies will have a resulting inflammatory reaction in their thyroid glands called "thyroiditis". Some cases manifest with a painful thyroid gland (sub-acute) while others do not (silent) but the majority of temporary thyroiditis conditions start with a phase of hyperthyroidism. Treatment for high levels of thyroid hormone is usually not necessary since the condition will resolve on its own over several weeks period of time. Treatment may only require bed rest and anti-inflammatory drugs for fever and thyroid inflammation.

Over-consumption of Iodine

People taking drugs that contain high-iodine content or who consume an excessive amount of iodine-rich foods such as kelp (seaweed) or supplements that contain higher-than-recommended daily allowances of iodine can cause hyperthyroidism to be induced.

In these cases, if the excessive iodine intake does not trigger an autoimmune response, causing permanent hyperthyroidism, the treatment would simply be to discontinue use of the products containing high levels of iodine.

Hot Nodules

Thyroid nodules are tumor-like growths that can develop within the thyroid gland. The majority of them do not affect thyroid hormone levels but a small percent can present as "hot nodules". This means the nodule has taken on features similar to thyroid gland tissue and is absorbing iodine coming into the body and producing thyroid hormones from it. This adds more thyroid hormone production to what the gland is already normally producing, causing the levels to become abnormally high.

Treatment for hot nodules may include surgical removal of them or removal of part of the thyroid gland (partial or sub-total thyroidectomy or lobectomy) or of the entire gland (total thyroidectomy).

Once thyroid tissue is removed via a corrective procedure, thyroid hormone replacement may also become necessary afterward, as a life long treatment.

Over-treated Hypothyroidism

Thyroid hormone replacement therapy is administered by an oral dose of T4 or combination T4 and T3 prescription thyroid hormone medication. The dose is then monitored through follow-up blood retests of the hormone levels in the patient's body. If a dose is too high and over-replacement is occurring, medication-induced thyrotoxicity can occur.

The treatment would be to reduce the patient's dose and to possibly stop the dose temporarily so that their thyroid hormone levels decrease back down into the normal values range.

Afterward the corrected dose-level would also need to be monitored via blood retests and at reasonable intervals throughout the patient's life.

Thyroid Autoimmunity

Graves' disease is the autoimmune cause of progressive hyperthyroidism in which auto-antibodies stimulate excessive production of thyroid hormones. Hashitoxicosis is also an autoimmune cause of hyperthyroidism but in this case, patients with Hashimoto's thyroiditis that typically causes progressive hypothyroidism (under-active) will first see the condition manifest with a phase of temporary hyperthyroidism.

Most patients experiencing Hashitoxicosis will not have additional flares of the condition once it initially resolves, although some do experience milder fluctuations in thyroid hormones due to flares of thyroiditis (phases of increased inflammation).

In rare cases, Hashimoto's thyroiditis will transition over to Graves' disease but most patients remain hypothyroid and require life-long thyroid hormone replacement therapy.

The Best Darn Hyperthyroidism Book!

Treatment for cases of hyperthyroidism from Graves' disease may include anti-thyroid drugs to reduce elevated thyroid hormone levels, beta-blocker medications to reduce hyperthyroid symptoms and possible eventual thyroid removal by surgery (thyroidectomy) or destruction of the gland by radioactive iodine (ablation).

CHAPTER THREE

Graves' Disease Hyperthyroidism and Treatments

Autoimmune Caused Hyperthyroidism

As mentioned in a previous chapter, Graves' disease is the leading cause of hyperthyroidism. Complications can include hypertension, cardiac arrhythmias and thyroid eye disease but treatments are available.

Graves' disease is an autoimmune condition affecting the thyroid gland that results in abnormally high levels of thyroid hormone to be released into the body causing hyperthyroidism. There is no cure for Graves' but progression of the disease can be halted by removing the thyroid gland. Mild to moderate cases may be successfully treated through drug therapies.

How Common is Graves' Disease?

Graves' disease affects up to 1% of the U.S. population or up to 3-million people.

This is about 5 in every 10,000 people and is 7 times more common in women than in men. Graves' patients are among the 190 million people worldwide who experience goiters but in the case of Graves' the goiter is "toxic" (toxic diffuse goiter), meaning it is causing abnormally high thyroid hormone levels or "thyrotoxicity" (hyperthyroidism).

Graves' patients can experience complications from the disease, including an inflammatory condition in the eyes called "Thyroid Eye Disease" or "Graves' Ophthalmology". It is estimated that about half (50%) of all Graves' patient will develop this complication of the disease affecting the eyes.

Is Hyperthyroidism Present in all Graves' Patients?

The point at which hyperthyroidism sets in varies among those found to have the auto-antibodies causing Graves' disease, called "Thyroid Stimulating Immunglobuin" (TSI).

Most patients may be positive for these "thyroid antibodies" months or years before the level of them becomes elevated enough to cause hyperthyroidism. The reason this may be the case is due to the fact that most people who are found to have Graves', are tested because they are already manifesting the signs or symptoms of hyperthyroidism. There are cases in which Graves' patients experience mild, early-onset goiters before their thyroid hormone levels become abnormally high.

Thyroid Antibodies common to both Graves' and Hashimoto's

The TSI are not the only antibodies present with Graves' but will co-exist with other thyroid antibodies that cause thyroid cell destruction, including the anti-thyroidperoxidase (Anti-TPO) and/or the anti-thyroglobulin (Anti-TG). These latter two mentioned antibodies are also present in Hashimoto's thyroiditis (autoimmune hypothyroidism) patients but are usually found in lower titers (positive lab measurements) in Graves' patients.

The Best Darn Hyperthyroidism Book!

Some Hashimoto's patients in fact are also found to be positive for TSI antibodies that typically cause Graves' but are in lower titers and may cause temporary hyperthyroid phases (Hashitoxicosis). These facts demonstrate how closely related these two autoimmune thyroid diseases are. It also offers explanation as to why some Graves' patients transition to Hashimoto's over time and the reverse has also been known to happen, although not common.

Symptoms and Treatment for Graves' Hyperthyroidism

When thyroid hormone levels have become abnormally high, causing the body's metabolism to become sped up, hyperthyroidism symptoms will develop. These include increased energy, nervousness and anxiety, rapid heart rate, hypertension, excessive sweating, diarrhea and weight loss. If Thyroid Eye Disease develops, the additional symptoms may include bulging, dryness, double vision (diplopia), and irritation of the eyeballs.

The Best Darn Hyperthyroidism Book!

Some cases of Graves'-caused hyperthyroidism are successfully treated with anti-thyroid drugs, which block thyroid hormone, reducing the amount entering the cells of the body and/or beta-blockers, which block the effects of epinephrine (adrenaline). When epinephrine is elevated in the body, it can cause cardiac arrhythmias and hypertension and elevated thyroid hormone levels speed up all bodily functions as a whole.

Determining which drug is needed or if a combination of them is needed, depends on how severe the hyperthyroidism is. Severe cases of Graves' hyperthyroidism that cannot be successfully treated with drug therapies may require surgical removal of the gland (thyroidectomy) or destruction of the gland using radioactive iodine (ablation).

Afterward, patients will need thyroid hormone levels corrected with replacement therapy.

The Best Darn Hyperthyroidism Book!

Treatment for Graves' Ophthalmology (Thyroid Eye Disease)

Thyroid Eye Disease (TED) is often treated using anti-inflammatory steroids (corticosteroids) to reduce inflammation, such as Prednisone. Eye drops may also be prescribed to keep dry eyes moistened. In cases when the disease is causing significant pressure on the optic nerve and presents the danger of vision loss, eye surgeries called "orbital radiotherapy" and/or "orbital decompression" may be necessary.

If eye protrusion is causing inability for a patient to close their eyes, surgery may be required to lengthen their eyelids. Many cases of TED have duration of from several months up to about 3 years and will improve spontaneously or with the aid of treatment depending on the severity.

Studies of TED have shown that Graves' patients who smoke more often experience TED or cases that are more severe.

CHAPTER FOUR

Radioactive Iodine Ablation of the Thyroid

Cell Destruction of Diseased Glands

This procedure abbreviated - RAI is performed by giving a patient an oral dose of radioactive iodine, which causes thyroid tissue death to cease its hyper-functioning.

RAI is the most commonly performed treatment for resolving cases of severe hyperthyroidism. Most people with Graves' disease, the most common cause of an overactive thyroid, are recommended for this procedure if medications fail to sufficiently slow-down an over-producing gland.

Patients with papillary or follicular thyroid cancer may also be referred for this procedure, following surgical removal of their glands (total thyroidectomy), to eradicate any remaining thyroid cells that can potentially contain malignancy.

How Does RAI Work?

The goal of RAI includes the following desired results:

- to destroy and eradicate all thyroid tissue and/or malignant cells in the body

- to stop the natural thyroid hormone production in the gland

- to correct hyperthyroidism

- to restore normal metabolism to the body

Once a dose of radioactive iodine that is large enough to completely kill the cells in a thyroid gland has been administered, the iodine is immediately absorbed by the gland. It does this because the thyroid is dependent on iodine to manufacture thyroid hormone. Once iodine enters the body through a person's diet or by oral dosing, the gland absorbs it to regulate bodily metabolism via these hormones.

An overactive thyroid gland will absorb more iodine than a normal-functioning gland will. Patients scheduled for RAI are placed on a "no iodine diet" for two weeks or more previous to the procedure, so that the thyroid gland absorbs the radioactive iodine as completely as possible.

What is the Result?

The radioactivity in the iodine enters the cells of the gland and causes them to die. The goal of the treatment is to fully eradicate all thyroid tissue from the body, so that it ceases to produce thyroid hormone. This will correct the hyperthyroidism.

Once thyroid hormone levels begin falling to lower levels following RAI, the overactive bodily metabolism slows down from the hyperthyroid state. Several weeks following the procedure the patient's thyroid hormone levels will fall to hypothyroid levels (under-active). The resulting hypothyroidism must be treated (usually lifelong) with thyroid hormone replacement.

The Best Darn Hyperthyroidism Book!

The hypothyroid therapy is administered to raise bodily metabolism back to a normal level.

What are the Risks?

RAI is a safe and effective procedure in most cases; there are, however, some medical sources that state that the treatment places some patients at risk for a worsening of thyroid eye disease (inflammatory condition in the eyeballs).

Other side effects that are temporary may include the following:

- sore throat

- dry mouth

- mild nausea

- dizziness

- fatigue

Some patients will rarely also see thyroid tissue that is not fully eradicated from the body that regrows and becomes revitalized and begins producing thyroid hormone. If it does so at an abnormally high level as it did before the procedure, this may require that the treatment be re-administered.

Patients are also required to be quarantined from family and pets for five to seven days due to risk of exposing them to radiation that remains in the body for a period following the procedure and can be spread by close contact.

Some thyroid-treating doctors offer a choice between thyroidectomy and RAI procedures to some of patients in need of thyroid ablation/removal (depending on individual cases). Patients should become educated about both options and fully discuss them with their treating doctor so that they feel comfortable and confident about the procedure they choose to have their doctors perform.

The Best Darn Hyperthyroidism Book!

CHAPTER FIVE

Treatment for Hashitoxicosis versus Graves' Disease

Patients with Temporary Hyperthyroidism

When Hashimoto's patients developing hypothyroidism, an under-active thyroid gland, go through "Hashitoxicosis", meaning temporary hyperthyroidism (overactive) they usually only register a slight difference in blood labs or only a mild indication of hyperthyroidism on them due to progressive hypothyroidism trying to take over. In other words, though these patients alternate between hyperthyroidism and hypothyroidism, it is temporary so that lab results of their thyroid hormone levels can at times be neutral or show only mild hyperthyroidism.

These patients may however test positive for "thyroid stimulating immunoglobulin" (TSI), the auto-antibody that typically contributes to Graves' disease (autoimmune hyperthyroidism).

The Best Darn Hyperthyroidism Book!

Once hypothyroidism does take over, they will need thyroid hormone replacement as a lifelong treatment. With Graves' disease, it settles in long enough to register as full blown hyperthyroidism on blood lab tests of thyroid hormone levels. This plus a high elevation of TSI antibodies can point to a definitive diagnosis of Graves' disease.

Rarely, Hashimoto's and Graves' can co-exist somewhat equally in a thyroid patient, so that they don't fully transition over to one or the other and when this occurs, the treatment may be destruction or surgical removal of the thyroid. Some countries treat these type patients that waver back and forth between the two disease, with a treatment called "block and replace" in which thyroid hormone blocking drugs (anti-thyroid) are first administered, followed by thyroid hormone replacement, once hypothyroidism has been fully induced. This treatment is rarely used in the USA .

Some doctors try an anti-thyroid drug or what's called a "PTU" (propylthiouracil and Carbimazole).

The Best Darn Hyperthyroidism Book!

This slows thyroid hormone production for Graves'-hyperthyroidism and after a trial of it, they will wean the patient off of it after a few months and see if the hyperthyroidism resolves. If not, they will then opt for RAI ablation (Radio Active Iodine destruction of the thyroid gland) or a thyroidectomy (surgical removal).

Many will first try a beta-blocker to see if it controls the hyperthyroid symptoms before going on to a PTU or a combination of the two.

If you are recommended for getting a thyroidectomy Vs RAI ask your doctor to go over the procedure with you (risks etc...), or to refer you to a doctor who can, so you can weigh the two options.

You might also ask him about anti-thyroid medications if he feels they are another possible option in your case. In short, I would say overt hyperthyroidism on blood lab test results definitely points to Graves' disease.

It is not that unusual for offspring of autoimmune thyroid disease parents to develop one or the other because the two diseases (Hashimoto's thyroiditis and Graves' disease) are more closely related than most people realize.

CHAPTER SIX

Why Doctors Sometimes Delay Treatment for Hashimoto's Thyroiditis

Problems with Hashitoxicosis

I created the article following below, from a response I wrote to a fellow thyroid patient experiencing severe anxiety symptoms with their Hashimoto's thyroiditis. I commented on this aspect of their thyroid disease case in the reply that follows.

My Reply:

Sometimes doctors are cautious about starting treatment due to the fact that if they treat when your thyroid hormones are fluctuating upward, which can happen earlier into the onset of Hashimoto's, they could cause you thyrotoxicity (hyperthyroidism). This would make anxiety symptoms even worse.

This fluctuation back and forth between hyper (overactive) and hypo (under-active) thyroid levels is common with autoimmune thyroiditis. When hyperthyroid phases are severe, it's called "Hashitoxicosis", so in my opinion, the doctor is wise in monitoring your case a while longer before starting you on thyroid hormone replacement. He likely will be blood retesting your levels at about 3-month intervals or so.

As far as treatment for anxiety symptoms, mine too were severe early into the onset of Hashimoto's thyroiditis and I personally used as-needed anti-anxiety drugs (like Xanax) but I did not use them for longer than a couple of months at a time and usually took half-doses rather than full ones. These type drugs (benzodiazepines) can be addictive and is why they should be taken with some caution. This is just an added option I would mention.

Also, you are absolutely right in that research studies state that Hashimoto's thyroiditis causes anxiety symptoms.

The Best Darn Hyperthyroidism Book!

Strangely there are doctors who do not have knowledge of that fact and will tell patients that the anxiety is not thyroid-related. In addition to medical studies, thousands of patients on forums, message boards and blogs attesting to having anxiety symptoms with Hashimoto's can't all be wrong! This is just lay-opinion but I would try low dose, as-needed anti-anxiety meds before accepting a prescription for the permanent daily-dosing type, such as SSRI antidepressants. There's nothing wrong with these and they can be greatly helpful when needed but your thyroiditis flares causing anxiety may diminish over a few months or even within a few weeks time, so starting a permanent regimen drug might be an over-kill so-to-speak at this point of observing your case. Certainly if emotional symptoms are severe or overwhelming and an as-needed drug is not helping enough, therapy can be very beneficial, as can permanent type drugs. I would never discourage any of these things when they are proven to be necessary.

:End of My Reply

CHAPTER SEVEN

Manifestations of Thyroid Eye Disease

Autoimmune Eyeball Problems and Their Treatments

Thyroid Eye Disease more commonly affects people with hyperthyroid conditions but can also occur in hypothyroid patients with thyroid autoimmunity.

Both inflammation and build up of fluid around the eyes can cause them to protrude (exophthalmos) and have an exaggeratedly wide-open appearance with Thyroid Eye Disease (TED), also referred to as "thyroid orbitopathy". The eyeball can also move forward from its position within the eye socket which can become severe in some cases (proptosis).

Patients with TED can experience dryness, redness and irritation within their eyes. A feeling of pressure and grittiness in the eyes can also occur, as well as difficulty with fully closing the eyelids.

The Best Darn Hyperthyroidism Book!

Treatments are available for this condition associated with cases of thyroid autoimmunity (diseases caused by thyroid antibodies).

Graves' Ophthalmopathy

Medical sources state that Graves' Ophthalmopathy is clinically apparent to varied degrees in up to 50% of Graves' disease patients, although other medical sources state that up to 80% of Graves' patients experience some type of eye symptoms as listed previously.

While Graves' is the autoimmune cause of thyrotoxicity, also referred to as "hyperthyroidism" TED can occur in approximately 10% of patients with the auto-antibodies that cause Grave's but whose thyroid hormone levels are euthyroid, meaning within normal values.

Only about 2% of Hashimoto's thyroiditis patients (those with autoimmune hypothyroidism) are affected by TED.

Optic Neuropathy

The optic nerves in the eyes of TED patients can also become affected due to their becoming compressed as a result of pressure from tissue-swelling in and around the eyeballs (orbital areas). With this condition that can be present with TED, a patient may experience pain, inability to see colors and/or partial loss of vision which will affect one or both eyes. Nerve cell damage may occur with optic neuropathy and eventual blindness is possible if treatment for TED is delayed.

The Role of Myxedema in TED

Myxedema is a term meaning tissues in the body are retaining fluid (edema) and a build-up of mucin (mucus) will cause a thickening of the skin in areas of the body, or what is also referred to as "pretibialmucinosis". The condition is often present in autoimmune thyroid disease patients who are experiencing TED. Areas on the face can become swollen for example and will have a puffy appearance.

The deep tissues around the eyes can also become swollen as well as tissues behind the eyes. This causes less area in the eye-sockets for movement and to retain the orbital position of the eyes, causing them to be pushed forward and to protrude.

Treatments for TED

The first line of treatment when TED is diagnosed is to correct any thyroid hormone imbalance that might be present if it is not already being done. In cases when thyroid autoimmunity is the cause of hyperthyroidism, patients may need to have their thyroid glands removed.

Some medical research studies state that surgical removal of the gland (thyroidectomy) may be a better choice than destruction of the gland by radioactive iodine (ablation) because of the risk the latter mentioned procedure may present to some patients with TED, in worsening the condition.

The following list of treatments may also be administered individually or in combination as determined by a treating physician.

• Prescription eye drops for added lubrication to help prevent dryness and redness.

• Corticosteroid (cortical steroid) and/or topical hydrocortisone to reduce inflammation in the eyes and in tissues surrounding the eyes.

• Radiotherapy or Decompression Surgery (possibly both) to reduce pressure in the eyeballs and to prevent potential damage to them.

• Surgery for lengthening the eyelids that do not fully cover the eyes due to protrusion of them.

• TED patients who are smokers can benefit by quitting due to chemicals in cigarettes that cause inflammation in the eyes and may also be a recommendation by their doctors.

The Best Darn Hyperthyroidism Book!

CHAPTER EIGHT

Symptoms and Manifestations of Thyroid Storm

The Hyperthyroid Condition Requiring Emergency Care

Thyroid Storm is a condition in which a thyroid patient experiences sudden, severe hyperthyroidism that requires emergency treatment to prevent injury or death.

This disorder of extremely severe hyperthyroid symptoms is rare but due to its potential to cause bodily injury through damage to organs and possible coma or death, all thyroid patients should have general knowledge about signs and symptoms of Thyroid Storm.

Symptoms

The symptoms of Thyroid Storm will occur suddenly and with extreme force. They are the symptoms of hyperthyroidism but some of the manifestations of the condition are not typical of common overactive thyroid conditions.

The Best Darn Hyperthyroidism Book!

The general symptoms of severe hyperthyroidism include very rapid heart (tachycardia), extreme nervousness and anxiety, chronic diarrhea, uncontrollable energy, severe hypertension and muscle weakness.

The non-typical symptoms of Thyroid Storm that occur with other severe hyperthyroid symptoms include mental confusion, psychosis (hallucinations and delusions), severe vomiting, unusual behaviors, a sudden high fever, heart arrhythmias that can progress to cardiac arrest and fainting spells.

These less common symptoms are likely the ones that would point to something beyond a phase of typical hyperthyroidism.

When these signs and symptoms appear, the patient should be taken into emergency medical care immediately, to prevent coma and/or death from occurring.

Is Thyroid Storm Exclusive to Hyperthyroid Patients?

No, the condition can also occur in hypothyroid patients although it is more common in those with hyperthyroidism, especially the autoimmune-caused type called Graves' disease. Patients with hypothyroidism caused by Hashimoto's (autoimmune thyroiditis) have also been known to experience Thyroid Storm and those patients who experience intermittent phases of hyperthyroidism referred to as "Hashitoxicosis" are at higher risk for having a Thyroid Storm.

Causes and Triggers

When Thyroid Storm occurs, the T3 and T4 thyroid hormones elevate to very high levels, causing severe thyrotoxicity (toxic levels). Graves' disease patients and others who are being treated for hyperthyroidism can experience Thyroid Storm if they suffer a heart attack or a severe infection in their bodies.

Any traumatic experience can result in this condition of severe hyperthyroidism, including accidents that cause severe physical trauma. Patients treated for hypothyroidism can experience the condition, if they are given excessively high levels of thyroid hormone replacement that causes their T4 and/or T3 levels to elevate far above normal values.

Treatments

The treatments for Thyroid Storm include those that are typical for treating hyperthyroidism but in this case the drugs that are administered must be done at higher doses until symptoms are brought under control. If a hyperthyroid patient has already received treatments to shut down their own thyroid hormone production (thyroid removal) and they are taking thyroid hormone therapy, the replacement hormone must be discontinued while treatment is given.

The treating physician will increase or begin administering levels of anti-thyroid drugs (to reduce thyroid hormone levels).

The Best Darn Hyperthyroidism Book!

Beta-blocker medications that calm hypertensive and cardiac arrhythmia symptoms might also be started. Anti-inflammatory drugs may also be needed to reduce inflammation and fever levels. This may include powerful corticosteroids (steroid anti-inflammatory) and/or over-the-counter drugs that reduce inflammation. Patients are closely monitored until symptoms of Thyroid Storm have diminished and there is no danger of relapse.

CHAPTER NINE

My Review of Mary Shomon's Hyperthyroid Book

Another Great Resource for Patients with Hyperthyroidism

Mary J. Shomon's book "Living Well with Graves' Disease and Hyperthyroidism" is a complete and thorough resource to help educate patients being treated for overactive thyroid glands of all causes, including Graves' Disease, which is the number one cause of hyperthyroidism worldwide.

(A special thanks to Mary for the review copy provided to me for this review.)

I appreciate the fact that Mary authored a book specifically for hyperthyroid patients and others who wish to learn about this thyroid disease, rather than simply including a detailed section for it in one of her other thyroid subject books.

The Best Darn Hyperthyroidism Book!

She could have easily done this with the fact that hypothyroid (under active thyroid) patients outnumber those with hyperthyroid conditions by about five to one. I believe this demonstrates her passion for providing thorough, quality information for hyperthyroid patients who also wish to live well with their disease. This book helps these patients to achieve and gain back as much quality-of-life as possible as treated hyperthyroid patients.

She addresses in detail the signs and symptoms of hyperthyroidism, including those physical ones caused by an abnormally increased metabolism in the body. She also addresses those signs of bodily changes, including goiter (thyroid swelling), nodules (tumors on/in the gland), hair loss and weight loss as well as the emotional symptoms of anxiety and depression. Co-morbid conditions caused by hyperthyroidism and Graves' are also discussed, including eye inflammation (Graves ' Ophthalmopathy) and skin related problems (Graves ' Dermopathy).

She continues with a chapter on the vastly important subject of getting diagnosed so that treatment for relieving symptoms and to begin healing in the body can be administered by a qualified Doctor. A chapter on integrative and holistic treatments is also included in addition to discussions on conventional medical treatments.

Mary also takes a detailed look at the medical tests used to diagnose hyperthyroid conditions, including common blood tests of thyroid hormone levels and imaging tests that detect toxic goiter and hot nodules that may contribute to overproduction of hormone by the thyroid gland. She also discusses the subject of "thyroid antibodies" with special emphasis on the auto-antibody most commonly associated with Grave's called "Thyroid Stimulating Immunoglobulin" (TSI).

In her thoroughness in covering these subjects related to hyperthyroidism, she also covers aspects relating to breastfeeding, infants, children and teens who, are affected.

The Best Darn Hyperthyroidism Book!

Also covered is the subject of post treatment hypothyroidism (low thyroid hormone) that requires treatment with thyroid hormone replacement therapy following removal or destruction of the gland in patients who require these type treatments.

I highly recommend this wonderful book to my readers who suffer hyperthyroidism, to those who suspect they may have an overactive thyroid and to anyone who is simply interested in a detailed study on all the important aspects of this serious but treatable thyroid condition. Patients can in fact live well with this disease and Mary Shomon has provided a great resource in helping patients to achieve this goal.

CHAPTER TEN

Support for Struggling Thyroid Patients

Two Reasons Why Information and Support Resources are Important

1. Newly diagnosed thyroid patients often express the fact that despite quality treatment for thyroid disease, their doctors do not have the ability due to time-constraints, to fully inform them about their disease/disorder.

Most patients feel a great need to understand what is happening to them (self-education) because the unknown aspects of thyroid problems can create fear and frustration in many patients.

2. Thyroid patients experience serious bouts of emotional issues from thyroid disease (anxiety and/or depression) and from the realities of experiencing the onset of a disease that will affect them, for the rest of their lives.

The Best Darn Hyperthyroidism Book!

A source of emotional support, such as a doctor, is not available to a patient, at any time a need might arise but only for a few minutes, at office visits that are relatively infrequent. Patients can feel very alone with their disease and even those closest to them, may be at a loss for knowing how to support and comfort them. --

The facts addressed in these two points alone help to point out the purpose and importance for the availability of information and support resources, that can be shared between thyroid patients. Fellow-patients can often relate better to each other than they can to their own healthy family members.

It is unfortunate when patients are told that they should not look into support resources online because they "might be led astray with wrong information" and that they should somehow rely solely on their doctor, not only for treatment but also for needed, general education about their disease and the often-needed support for coping with it.

Getting these needs met by a treating doctor is simply not possible in most cases, unless a patient's spouse or close relative is a doctor. In the case of a patient who doesn't especially feel the need for information and support, it wouldn't be necessary to begin with but for many patients it can actually mean survival if they are seriously affected by their disease. It is sometimes forgotten that complications from thyroid disease can include things such as Thyroid Eye Disease, Obstructive Goiters, chronic mood disorders and Thyroid Storm (potentially life threatening).

Most thyroid patients have the common sense to learn from reputable sources when doing an online search about their disease and to the compare information they find with other reliable sources, so that it is confirmed. At many thyroid disease forums and message boards for example, patients share general information that can be confirmed by reputable source-links, plus they can offer support that comes from fellow-patient experience.

The Best Darn Hyperthyroidism Book!

To deny patients this type help, for fear of them being led astray by incorrect information etc..., could mean tremendous lost opportunities for patients who have serious struggles coping with their thyroid disease.

CHAPTER ELEVEN

Coping with Thyroid Disease

Methods for Dealing with a Lifetime Health Disorder

Educate Yourself about your Thyroid Disorder

Being newly diagnosed with a thyroid disease or disorder can be concerning and can sometimes create more anxiety in a person when they feel less informed about what is happening to them.

Doctors do not always have enough time to thoroughly educate their patients about their diagnosis due to having large numbers of patients to treat as mentioned previously. Some doctors help educate their patients by providing them with informative brochures about their thyroid conditions.

In addition to information your doctor provides, you can also search online for information that will help generally educate you.

The Best Darn Hyperthyroidism Book!

Reputable and reliable sources are a great way to become better informed about symptoms, treatment and any risks for developing other related problems from your thyroid disorder. Some of the better thyroid information sources include the AACE (American Association of Clinical Endocrinologists), MedLinePlus (National Institutes of Health), WebMD and the ATA (American Thyroid Association).

Join Fellow Patient Thyroid Forums and Support Groups

You can get connected to other thyroid patients by joining forums and groups that offer support to thyroid patients. Many of these forums are volunteer and non-profit. Others do make money from ad space they sell or share but many times this is to help run the forum or group they moderate or administrate and to cover any expenses.

By corresponding with other thyroid patients through these types of resources, you can hear their personal stories.

You may possibly relate-to many of the things they struggle with in regard to symptoms. You may also hear pointers for getting the best possible treatment for optimal recovery of your health and a better quality of life. There are a number of thyroid forums available, but two of the more reputable are the MedHelp International and HealthBoards thyroid disease forums.

Be Proactive in your Treatment and become a Partner with your Doctor

This simply means you are advocating representing yourself in getting the best possible treatment for your thyroid disease from your doctor. This is better accomplished by first becoming educated about your thyroid disease as mentioned in step one above. A doctor must hear as much as they can from their patient because we are the only person who can let him know how well our treatment is relieving our symptoms.

Doctors are also usually open to suggestions from patients who may feel they need a certain test run to better evaluate how well their treatment is going or in suggesting a change in the dose-level of a medication they are receiving. Of course this type partnering needs to be done in balance so that your doctor doesn't feel that you are not placing trust in him in administering proper treatment. Your goal is simply to help him know how your treatment is going and what you would reasonably like to see accomplished for you over time.

Help to Educate other Thyroid Patients

By referring fellow patients to helpful resources you have received a benefit from and by sharing your personal story you can help to educate them. Sharing the same type of support you have received can serve as a type of therapy in your own continued coping as well. Some thyroid patients, such as me, will begin to compose articles in contributing toward fellow patient education by helping share helpful and general information.

The Best Darn Hyperthyroidism Book!

This type of help is sometimes referred to as "Thyroid Patient Advocacy" because the advocate helping fellow patients is also a thyroid patient. Some patients relate better to those who are going through the same or similar experience than they can to their healthy family members or even their own doctors. Doctors can be excellent at treating thyroid diseases, but when it comes to support and coping, fellow patients can sometimes be the best source.

If you are a struggling or a newly diagnosed thyroid patient, consider searching online for helpful information, support and sources that can help you better-cope and regain a better quality of life.

It is my hope that this book is a resource that contributes toward that goal for many thyroid patients and I extend my sincere appreciation and best wishes to each reader!

(END)